Have Your Cake…

And Look Good Too!

By: Eric Knight Jr.

Table of Contents

Intro

Your life is terrible because you eat meat and meat bi-products. Everything that's wrong with the world is because you aren't vegan. Have you ever felt like this is the message that the rest of the world is sending you?

I know I have. Don't get me wrong, there is nothing wrong with someone deciding to adopt a vegan, vegetarian, or whatever type of eating lifestyle you want, but what is wrong is when someone else tries to make you feel like dirt because you don't choose 'their' way.

I love broccoli, but I also love steak. I

absolutely adore fresh fruit, but I also love fresh baked chocolate chip cookies.

I can hear some of you saying *"But my personal trainer says that I need to eat 10 small vegan meals a day!"*. I have done some training and I have helped numerous people come up with eating plans. This allows me to know many personal trainers, and guess what... almost every one I know has a different philosophy when it comes to what and how you should be eating.

One will tell you that dairy is completely off limits and that soy is a much better alternative. Then the next one will tell you that whey (dairy) is the superior protein and soy is horrible for you.

One says that you should only eat 1 big meal a day and the other says that you should eat 7 small meals a day.

I could keep going but I believe you get it. My point is there are several different ways to get into great shape on both the inside and the outside, and anyone who tells you otherwise is closed minded, ignorant, or both.

All of this led me to ask a question that changed my life in regards to staying in pretty good shape.

The question is ***"If I am not a body builder, a fitness model, or a professional athlete, why do I***

have to eat like one?"

The answer is you don't.

Before I tell you about the eating plan that allowed me to enjoy ALL of the foods that I liked and still stay in good/great shape, I need to give a disclaimer.

***TIP** If your Dr. has you on a special diet or you already have existing medical conditions, consult your medical professional before you make any special changes. Ok, let's go.

I love good food, therefore, I had to come up with something that would not only allow me to <u>get</u> into great shape, but to <u>stay</u> in great shape, all the while enjoying the foods I really like. Many people said that my goal was impossible, but I didn't buy that. I accomplished my goal and now I am going to share my (anti-diet) plan with you.

The Plan

The first step in my plan was to identify the enemies of your having the body you want. Actually, there are 4 enemies: 1. Bad Fats, 2. Bad Carbs, 3. Extra Sugar, 4. High Sodium. (Reducing the enemies also cuts calories because most calories come from carbs and fats.)

If you have ever tried a diet that required you to completely cut the 4 enemies out, then you know how difficult it is to do. Attempting to cut sodium alone is ridiculously hard (not to mention removing sodium completely makes food taste terrible).

Let me tell you what I did. I knew that completely getting rid of salt, sugar, carbs, and fat wasn't a realistic option for me, but what I could do was greatly reduce those things, and add other healthy foods to my day to day diet.

The first thing I did was probably the simplest thing someone could do to have a positive effect on their body.

1. I started drinking more water.

Many sources will tell you that you should drink half of your body weight in ounces (oz.) of water, a day. That is not a realistic option for many people. Many who are working to lose weight are severely overweight. Let's say that a person is 400 lbs. It is not likely that they will able to drink 200 oz. of water a day, especially if they have a job. They would be going to the restroom an obscene amount of times a day. What worked for me is a minimum of 64 oz. of water a day. My goal was 100 oz. a day (96 oz. rounded up), but my minimum was 64 oz.

You need water for so many reasons that I won't even attempt to name them all, but there are a few that pertain to this eating plan. One of the reasons water is important is because adequate amounts of water help us flush the body of toxins.

You can't flush without water, and an accumulation of toxins can cause all kinds of havoc in the body.

Water also helps the body dilute and flush sodium. That will help you with the sodium levels in your body. You do need sodium as it is an essential mineral, but too much can lead to high blood pressure and other issues.

2. The next thing I did was what I call the

'Sugar Draft'

I really liked candy and sodas, but I liked cookies, cakes, brownies, and pies/pastries even more. So what I did was I picked the 4 or 5 types of sweet foods I absolutely loved and I got rid of the rest. I didn't cut out all sugar, but I became very selective about my sugar intake.

I was super picky about where I was getting my sugar from. When I said "where I was getting my sugar from", I didn't mean the location, I meant the food. I liked candy, but it pretty much all had to go because it didn't make the cut when I did my draft. The only candy I continued to eat was Snickers, and that wasn't an everyday thing.

That was it for candy. I also cut sodas completely. As much as I loved them, they had to go because they are just empty calories and carbs. Empty calories are calories that come with no nutritional value. If you look at the nutritional label on the side of soft drinks, you will see that they have little to no vitamins or minerals (no health benefits). That is what makes them empty calories. Cutting sodas and most candy reduced my sugar intake drastically. The sugar that I was eating was going to be something that I really enjoyed.

Now when I eat cookies and cake, it doesn't affect me nearly as much because I cut the sugar in so many other areas, but I took it a step further. If you don't know it, homemade foods are typically much healthier than store bought foods and most restaurant foods. Scratch made foods are even better. Why?

Because foods that are pre-made tend to

have preservatives and things to make the food look fresh even though it could have been prepared months ago. Food dye/coloring is an example of something unhealthy that is often added to food to make it look fresh. The producers of these products don't often care a lot about your health, but they do care about money. So what they end up doing is packing products with tons of inexpensive bi-products that make foods last longer, but they are terrible for our bodies.

Knowing all of this, I decided to select only the sweets that I really liked, and I was only going to eat them if I made them myself. I could go out and buy a cake every week, but I knew I wasn't going to bake a cake every week... but even if I did bake one every week, it would be much healthier than me buying one because I would only use real ingredients at home. My cake would only have flour, eggs, sugar, vanilla, and other real foods. It wouldn't be like that super long list of ingredients on some store bought products.

A quick recap in a nutshell is that I gave up nearly all sweets (and sodas) that weren't homemade cookies, brownies, pie, and cake. I didn't waste my sugar intake. I only used it on the homemade sweets that I really loved.

Cutting those things out greatly reduced my sugar, fat, and carb intake, which in turn lowered my caloric intake.

Ok, that's enough of what I stopped doing, now let's get to some of the habits that I added to my eating.

We already talked about me making sure that I was drinking a minimum of 64oz. of water a day. 3. I also added more fresh fruits and both cooked and fresh vegetables to my daily diet.

Many people feel like eating healthy is too expensive, and that is partly true, but these days fresh fruits and vegetables such as lettuce, broccoli, and apples can be purchased at low prices, especially if you catch them on sale. Some stores have great sales on their produce. You just have to shop around.

Fresh fruits and vegetables supply your body with valuable nutrients and fiber, both of which help with weight loss and overall health. Do your best to eat some type of fresh veggies or fruits with every meal.

Fruits and vegetables are also great as snacks. It does you no good to change most of your eating habits and then ruin your results with terrible snacking. Unhealthy snacks can destroy your progress.

One of my favorite snacks is freshly popped popcorn. You may not know this, but popcorn is actually a very healthy snack...if you cook it yourself and don't load it up with butter, oil, or any other unhealthy topping. I love movie popcorn as much as anyone you will ever meet, but I save my movie popcorn for the movies. Keep in mind that I don't even go to the movies every month. Some people go multiple times a month.

If that is you, then you probably shouldn't get buttered popcorn every time you go, but if you go every now and again like I do, then you will probably be fine enjoying the movie style popcorn barring any health issues. But when I am at home, I don't attempt to make my popcorn the way I like it at the movies. The healthy ways are to pop your kernels in a small amount of oil on the stove-top, or to get an air popper (You could even use olive oil if you like.), then salt it to taste while the corn is still hot. You could add other seasonings if you like, but make sure that what you add is not unhealthy.

If you think microwave popcorn is a healthy option, think again. Microwave popcorn tends to have lots of oil and often times food coloring. Even if you cook your popcorn in oil, it will likely not be as oily as microwave popcorn. Don't just take my word for it. Look at the nutrition facts on microwave popcorn vs. the facts on the bottle or bag of un-popped kernels. You will likely find that the un-popped kernels have nearly twice as much fiber and more protein than microwave popcorn with non of the artificial flavorings or colors.

Ok. Let's recap everything that I added to my eating plan.

-The first thing was a minimum of 64oz of water.

-I made sure to try to add vegetables (mostly green) or fresh fruits to every meal.

-I made sure to utilize healthy snacks such as freshly popped popcorn, fresh fruit, fresh vegetables, and nuts.

The final step I took really helped me to achieve and maintain my results. I found a healthy meal replacement shake.

Meal Replacement Shakes

Yes, you read that correctly. Notice that I said a *meal replacement shake* and not a protein shake. Many people seem to think that they are the same thing but they are not. A meal replacement shake should have many of the things that you should get in a healthy meal, and that includes protein.

-A protein shake might have a few vitamins and minerals, but they are typically all about the protein.

-Meal replacement shakes tend to have a lot more nutrition (vitamins, minerals, and other nutrients) and fiber.

I found a meal replacement shake that had not only the nutrition I wanted, but it was low carb, low fat, low sugar, and low sodium. It tasted pretty good too. The truth is there are several meal replacement shakes out there, but they are not all created equal. What I recommend is that you find a shake with no artificial sweeteners, colors, or anything else... if you can find one.

Let me warn you. It is super difficult to find a good tasting, natural meal replacement shake. Nearly every meal replacement shake on the market contains the artificial sweetener sucralose. In fact, the very first meal replacement shake that I used to get in shape contained sucralose. It is said that sucralose is "the best" of the artificial sweeteners, but it is still artificial, so try to avoid it if possible.

(I know many of you are diabetic and probably already use sucralose because you can't have very much sugar. If that is what you have to do, then do that. Do what is best for you.)

The other side of the delicious all natural shake is the price. If you happen to find one, they are probably going to charge you 3 arms and a leg. I am just warning you so that you are prepared for the hunt. But don't worry too much because they do exist.

I don't want to sound too pessimistic because there actually are good tasting shakes that don't require you to re-finance your house. I found one so I know that you can too.

Keep in mind that another benefit of a M.R.S. is that it is replacing a meal, so if you break it down, even an expensive one could be $6 a meal. That is cheaper than the meals many people buy.

It's important that you find an effective shake that you like because your shake is a huge part of what we do to get the results we desire.

Enjoying Foods You Like While Getting/Staying In Shape

There is a debate among many people in the fitness industry about how many meals a day a person should eat. Some say you should eat 6-10 small meals a day, while some believe it is best to eat 1 huge meal a day. I have never seen anything to make me believe that any one way is best for every one. I personally stick to 3 meals a day because it works well for this plan. This whole plan is about being healthy and in pretty good shape while still being able to enjoy the foods we really like.

Many eating plans aren't sustainable for most people because most people aren't body builders or figure models, therefore, most people aren't likely to give up gooey brownies with cool ice cream on top or crispy and juicy, perfectly fried chicken. If you are like me, it is going to have to be life or death before I stop eating pepperoni pizza.

So the question is how do you eat these delicious foods and lose weight at the same time?

Let me tell you my whole story.

In 2010 I had a job in a building that had a

free gym for the employees. I was in pretty good shape, but I was thicker than I preferred. At that point I was the most consistent I had ever been in regards to working out, but I couldn't get a flat stomach to save my life. Then they let me go from my job so I lost access to the gym.

Needless to say, my physique suffered greatly. I found out about a meal replacement shake that was helping people get pretty good results. I saw several before and after pictures of people who had both lost weight and added lean muscle. The shake was loaded with nutrition and fiber, and I was down to try a meal replacement shake, because outside of the fact that my physique was going down the tubes, I often have a problem deciding what I want to eat, especially for breakfast. I thought a meal replacement could help with that and I was right.

There are typically 2 main ways to utilize meal replacement shakes.

Option 1- You replace 1 meal a day and eat actual food (preferably healthy food) for your other 2 meals.

This option is typically for people who don't get to eat breakfast, don't have time to eat lunch, or just want to add lean muscle. If the shake is nutritious like it should be, this is also a good way to get extra nutrition in your system.

Option 2- You replace 2 meals and eat normal food for your remaining meal. Most good meal replacement shakes will be lower in sugar, fat, and sodium than the foods people typically eat. So replacing 2 meals is generally great for losing weight and leaning out if the shake has a high quality protein. If the protein is of high quality, you won't need the astronomical amounts that body builders use. The shakes I used have about 12 grams of protein per meal.

Many people would have looked at me and felt that I was fine the way I was and that I didn't need to lose any weight, but I had a gut forming and I had to nip that quickly. I wanted to lean out.

I decided to replace 2 meals a day and I ate whatever I wanted for my other meal. 2 things happened that absolutely blew my mind. The 1st thing was I had a nagging shoulder injury that had been getting progressively worse for about 6 months. When I implemented my shakes, my shoulder pain was at it's peak. Two weeks or so after I started my shakes, my shoulder pain was considerably better, and a month later my shoulder wasn't hurting at all.

Was it the shake?...Yes and no.

I give the credit to answered prayers and nutrition. The shake was just the vehicle that carried the nutrition. I firmly believe that I could have taken a great vitamin supplement and gotten the same results as far as my shoulder goes. ***Cranking up your nutrition can have all types of unexpected benefits on your health.***

The 2nd thing that happened completely blew me away. Let me give a little more back story. I told you earlier that I worked out at my job, but even then I couldn't get a flat stomach. I had been working out the majority of my adult life, and I was never able to get rid of it. Even when I was skinny, I still had the 'pooch' at the bottom of my abs. I ran, played basketball, lifted weights, and did hundreds of reps on the ab machine and the 'pooch' wouldn't budge.

Once I started replacing my 2 meals a day and eating whatever I wanted for the 3rd meal (I don't do a lot of snacking), it took about 2 weeks for the 'pooch' to be gone. **I had a flat stomach with no working out.**

I hadn't worked out for 6 months due to the shoulder injury, so you can imagine my shock when I got a flat stomach at a time when I couldn't work out at all. I could only imagine the results I would get once I was able to work out in conjunction with my meal plan. I didn't want to be stupid and re-injure myself, so I waited for a few months even though my shoulder no longer hurting. 120 or so days later, I found out what type of results I would get.

I was absolutely elated with my results. Before that point, I never believed that I could achieve those types of results... and that was only the beginning.

So again, I was replacing 2 meals a day with my shakes and I was eating whatever I wanted for my 3rd meal. My non-shake meal could be anything from pizza to tacos or maybe pancakes, and this was before I started working out.

There are many personal trainers who will tell you that this is impossible.

I know many great, open-minded trainers who are only concerned with getting you results, but some trainers are self-righteous know-it-all's who believe that their way is the only way.

There are likely several ways for you as a non-body builder to accomplish your physical fitness goals, but I believe using meal replacements is the best way for most people.

Why?

I am glad you asked.

Nutrition

I want to make sure that I begin this section by telling you that I am not a doctor, nor do I want to come to you from that perspective. What I do want to do is explain what nutrition is and why it is important through my own experiences.

Through out my journey of balancing being healthy with enjoying life, I've learned that many (if not most) people don't care very much about nutrition or their health. Let me tell you what made me focus nutrition, and therefore health.

Back around 2005 I was working 3rd shift and something happened that had never happened to me before. I was driving home on the interstate doing approximately 60 miles per hour. It was around 3 or 4 in the morning and I felt like the only one on the road. I was in the center of 3 lanes, and then I blinked. Well, I thought I blinked, but apparently I closed my eyes and went to sleep for around a min.

When I opened my eyes, I was coming up on the next exit, which was a mile away from the last thing I remembered seeing. Thank God for Grace because I was still in the center lane.

I had been having trouble sleeping since high school, but up until that point, it hadn't been a problem. I had never come close to going to sleep behind the wheel before. That scary experience was a wake-up call. I knew I had to do something because if things had been a little different, I wouldn't be here today to tell this story.

But there was another problem... I had no idea why I couldn't sleep. I would be so tired and sleepy but I either couldn't fall asleep or I would wake up in the middle of sleep. After a lot of thought and deliberation, I came to the conclusion that I must have been missing something that my body needed. I was missing some essential vitamin or mineral. In other words, I needed more nutrition.

Although I had determined that I was deficient in something, I had no idea what that something was, so I began taking your typical brand name, off the grocery store shelf vitamin and mineral supplements. I took them for a while, but I didn't notice any type of improvement.

I wasn't about to give up, so I started doing research and I learned that not all supplements are created equal, even if the listed amounts of vitamins and minerals are the exact same. Some supplements have higher quality ingredients or better absorption rates. I began to try different products from sources people might not think of trying. I knew that direct sales companies often times have higher quality products than you can get from a store, so I began to check into some of those.

The first supplements I got were night and day better than the “brand name' supplements I bought. I not only got better sleep, but I felt much better all around. Even though I was better, I still wasn't getting the kind of sleep I should have been getting. The good news was although I hadn't achieved the types of results I was seeking,

I knew I was on the right track. I began to try all of the supplements, super foods, and nutritional juices I could find, and at the end of the search, I was sleeping better, had more energy, and my troublesome skin began to clear up.

Sleeping better was definitely the biggest thing. My ability to get good sleep is now my barometer for deciding if a supplement is good or not. If I tried a new supplement and I was not sleeping well after 90 days max, I would feel like it wasn't the one for me. So this is how nutrition became a huge part of my life.

One thing I noticed while I was doing my

research was how complicated many outlets made nutrition sound. If you tried to find out what nutrition was and why it should matter to you, you likely would have come away more confused and with even more questions than you had before you started. When I explain nutrition, I try to do it in a way that is simple to understand.

Think of your body as a car and nutrition as the gas, or quality of gas that you put into your car. Have you ever had bad gas in your car? If you haven't had the luxury of putting bad gas in your car then you might not fully appreciate this example.

Bad gas will make your car do all sorts of strange

things that you would never think gas could affect. When a car has bad gas, it (the car) will perform like a piece of trash, and when it has good gas, it runs great. There is a reason most high tech engines and luxury cars require high octane premium gas.

Similarly, our bodies perform like trash when all they get is bad food, or not enough nutrition. We should be getting the fuel for our bodies (nutrition) from the food we eat. Have you ever asked yourself the question "why do we eat?" ? Many people feel like we eat 'to get full'. We definitely don't want to starve, but getting full isn't the primary reason to eat.

The primary reason to eat is to get nutrition/nutrients into our bodies. The word nutrition is derived from a Latin word meaning 'to feed' or 'nourish'. What do we call a person who hasn't had enough to eat?... malnourished. Therefore you could have a full belly and still be malnourished because having a full belly doesn't mean your body has a sufficient amount of nutrients. It's like you can be drinking liquids yet still be dehydrated.

This is why people can experience a number of health benefits when they increase their nutritional intake. Many ailments occur because our bodies are deficient in something that we need but aren't getting, but when we start getting these nutrients, things can sometimes turn around. I am not saying that nutrition is going to heal you if you have a disease, but I am saying that you never know what results you might get when you increase your nutrition.

Typically, the higher your nutrition intake, the better you feel, and your overall health improves. The fact is that the body is a more efficient machine when we give it the proper nutrition. Hopefully this gives you a better idea of why nutrition is important to your overall health and why it is an important part of this eating plan.

Why Do Meal Replacements Work?

You are probably wondering how it is possible that you can eat foods like pizza and fried chicken along with shakes and still lose weight. It actually makes complete sense why it works so well.

Depending on how active you are, most sources will recommend that you get around 2000 calories a day. If you aren't very active, then you might not need 2000 and if you are very active, you could need more than 2000, but 2k is the general number for most people.

If you are eating 3 meals a day, that averages out to 667 calories per meal to achieve your 2000 calories a day. If you eat something really lite for breakfast, like a large apple, that would be about 116 calories. If you subtract 116 from 2000, that leaves you with 1884 calories to split between the remaining 2 meals. Evenly split, that would leave 942 calories for lunch and 942 calories for dinner.

Let's say the apple you ate for breakfast was so good that you decided to have another along with a small turkey sandwich for lunch. That would equate to about 240 calories for lunch.

So you had 116 calories for breakfast, and 240 calories for lunch adding up to a total of 356 calories. If you subtract 356 from 2000, you still have 1644 calories for dinner. With the calories left over, you can eat nearly any type of food you want.

This isn't an eating recommendation. This is just an example to show you how the numbers work.

A quick side note on calories. Many people feel like calories are calories and that they are all equal. I am here to tell you that is not the case, especially when it comes to your overall health. If you recall, in the beginning I said that the 3rd enemy of you having the body you want is ‘extra’ sugar. What I meant by 'extra', or added sugar, was the granulated white sugar or brown sugar that you add to food and drinks.

I have a quick question for you... which would you say is the healthiest, a 115 calorie piece of fresh fruit or a 90 calorie small doughnut?

Many people feel as though the doughnut is healthier or better for losing weight simply because it is lower in calories.

I beg to differ.

Fresh fruit has natural sugar along with

vitamins and minerals while a doughnut has bad carbs from added sugar, fat, and flour, not to mention little to no nutritional value. Although fresh fruits and veggies might have more calories than many man made snacks, fruits and veggies are better for you. Many low calorie weight loss products are nutrient deficient meaning they have no real nutritional value.

This explains how you can stay in pretty good shape and health while still occasionally enjoying the foods you really like. When you change one or two of your meals to a good meal replacement shake, your caloric intake should work just like the example above, not to mention you should see and feel significant benefits because your nutritional intake should be much higher.

Some of you are probably thinking, “There is no way that I can replace 2 of my meals with shakes. I love food! I like to chew!” Let me ask you something... for those of you who eat 3 meals a day, how many of those 3 meals do you get to sit down and truly enjoy?

Many people don't eat breakfast at all, and lunch generally consists of what ever you can get and still make it back to work on time.

I don't know anyone who gets to sit and

fully enjoy all 3 meals everyday. Generally, the only meal people get to truly enjoy is dinner at home with the family. Many diets don't allow you to enjoy even that one meal and that is why many stop the diet and don't get to the point of making it a lifestyle change. Most diets are also inconvenient. A good meal replacement shake should be simple to quickly make in either a small blender or a shaker cup.

When you incorporate meal replacement shakes into your lifestyle, you can come home and eat pizza with the family instead of watching them eat pizza (or whatever food you love) while you eat something that you don't really want because it is supposedly healthy. Not being able to ever enjoy the foods you really want to eat while others eat those foods right in front of you is another reason why many people can't stick to a diet.

Don't get me wrong. If you want positive results, you must have some level of discipline.

Discipline

My advice is to move that discipline to something that you can do long term instead of something that you can only do temporarily.

Instead of using that discipline to completely avoid the foods you really like, use that discipline to avoid the sweets you don't really have to have or to make sure that you are getting at least 64 oz. of water a day. Speaking of discipline, use your discipline to drink your meal replacement shakes until your body adjusts and it becomes a habit.

Most types of physical change require some discomfort.

There are 2 things you should expect when you are starting a healthy journey, especially one that includes fiber and reducing your sugar. The first is the detox effect. If you have ever done any type of detox, then you are already familiar with detox side effects, but if you haven't done a detox, I want you to know what to expect. When your body gets the nutrition and fiber it needs, it begins to remove toxins from the body. Once toxins are pulled from the body, you could get skin breakouts, detox headaches, or gas.

The skin breakouts occur because the body is using your pores to help eliminate toxins. A detox headache is a mild headache that is usually around the front of the forehead. They can come and go randomly.

I would imagine you already know what gas is. It occurs due to getting the proper amount of fiber, but it usually goes away after your body adjusts.

In my experience, the detox side effects tend to last around 2 weeks max. They could last a little longer, or they could be shorter. I suppose it depends on your body's level of toxicity. The good news is once the side effects have passed, people generally report feeling better than they have in a long time, or ever.

That wraps up the detox effects. The next thing you should expect when starting your healthy journey that includes meal replacement shakes is the illusion of hunger. Allow me to clarify.

Shakes typically end up being 8-12 fluid ounces. If you take a glass of 8-12 fluid oz. of liquid and sit it beside a typical meal, you will likely find that the meal on the plate looks like a much larger meal than the liquid in the cup.

Since 8-12 ounces is so much smaller than the amount people typically eat, you might feel as though you need more to eat after you first start your meal replacements. If you have a high quality replacement, you should be getting everything you are supposed to get in a healthy meal, so no matter how you feel, you shouldn't be starving. It should actually be the complete opposite. Unless you are already a super healthy eater and you use supplements, you will likely be getting more nutrition from your shakes than you would from a regular meal anyway.

Keep this info in mind when you hit the mental hump that makes you think you need to eat a lot more. If you do eat something, make sure it is a healthy snack to hold you until your next meal.

When I first started, I found myself looking through the pantry although I wasn't really hungry.

If you are like me, you associate being full with a feeling. Shakes are smaller in mass, so you don't get that 'full feeling' you get with a heavy meal. Once you get used to not having that 'feeling', then it's smooth sailing. It only took me about 2 weeks to get used to not having that full feeling.

A big plus for those of you who are working to lose weight is the shakes will eventually help you to eat less. I am no Dr., but it's as though your stomach gets smaller because you are eating smaller meals. Your stomach doesn't need to expand as much (if at all) when you are taking in smaller meals.

The fiber and consistent water drinking help to sweep and flush the digestive tract leading to more productive bowel movements. Better bowel movements not only help you to remove toxins, but it also helps you to have a flatter stomach.

As you can see, a little discipline can help you to make changes to your health that you can sustain long term instead of having your health and weight bounce back and forth because of some unrealistic diet plan.

When the end result is true change, the one thing that can't be omitted (in any type of program) is discipline and sacrifice. The difference between programs is typically the amount of sacrifice required to see the program to success. Be very leery of anyone who tells you there is only one way to improve your health. There are several plans that can help you to lose weight and keep it off. There are several plans that can help you to add muscle. There are multiple ways to lower blood pressure and blood sugar.

The 2 questions you have to ask yourself

are ‘what sacrifices are you willing to make to achieve your desired result’, and ‘will you be able to sustain those sacrifices so that you can maintain those results long term’?

Some plans require you to cut out all carbs and fats. This is something that you shouldn't do for very long anyway, so it doesn't make a good long term solution. Some plans have you cut out all meats and meat bi-products such as milk and butter. These plans can be very effective for some people when it comes to improving health. There are many people who have seen positive results in regards to losing weight and improving their health numbers using a vegan or vegetarian plan.

The problem for many people is that outside of a life and death situation, cutting out all meats and sugar is not something that they are willing or able to do for a sustained amount of time (sometimes a life or death situation isn't even enough). I have seen many instances of people adopting a vegetarian diet and losing weight only to gain it all back a few months later because they didn't maintain the diet.

The reason I was/am able to stick to my eating plan for so long is not because it didn't require discipline, but because of where the discipline was applied. Allow me to explain.

Every good plan requires you to be disciplined in regards to consistency. If you don't do whatever the plan requires, then you can't expect to get the results the plan is supposed to deliver. Many plans and diets require you to be disciplined in completely giving up the foods you really like. That is a lot to ask of a person who isn't trying to be a body builder or a fitness model.

What makes the plan I used so simple and effective for most people is that your discipline needs to be directed towards being consistent with your meal replacements instead of never eating a piece of cake.

**If you are a drinker or a smoker, you will need a special type of discipline because you need to cut out the cigs and booze if you want to have positive health results.*

If you are responsible with your shakes and meal portions, you should see results barring any other health problem that could make it difficult for you to lose weight such as a thyroid issue. It's simple math. If you are taking in less calories while adding nutrition, you should see health improvements of some sort if you are currently overweight.

Adding Exercise And Physical Activity

If you really want to maximize your results, you could incorporate some form of working out. Nearly any program that focuses on improving your health will see increased results if some form of exercise is added to the program. This eating plan is no different.

Drinking more water, getting more protein, getting more nutrition, all while lowering bad carbs, calories, and fat is wonderful, but adding exercise will make it amazing. Anything you can do should help you get better results. If the most you can do is walk, that will help tremendously. If you incorporate a full exercise routine, you can get GREAT results.

I told you earlier how I got a flat stomach before I ever did any physical activity, and I couldn't wait until I could get back into the gym. I wasn't the Hulk or anything, but I never thought I could get the results that I achieved after only 90 days of working out on my plan.

I never thought I could have a 6 pack. 2 years later after maintaining my physique and medical numbers, I thought to myself "How far can I take this… What kind of results can I really achieve?”.

So I decided to dedicate 90 days to getting in the best shape of my life... again. This time I ramped everything up. I increased my cardio and I switched my gym schedule from every other day for 3 days to 5 days straight with 2 days of rest. I also incorporated an “Insane” work out DVD program. Most of my life I was a small and skinny kid who was almost always looked over. I never imagined that I could be in good enough shape that other people would ask me to help them get into shape, but that is exactly what happened.

Hopefully my results encourage you and let you know that if you stick to a good plan, then the sky is the limit. You don't want to be on a diet, you want a plan that you can use to get in shape and stay in shape instead of yo-yoing back and forth. It worked for me and it can work for you too.

How I Made My Shakes Work For Me

If you don't eat breakfast at all, eat a high fat, high carb, no nutrition fast food lunch, and a high fat, high carb, no nutrition fast food dinner that totals 3000 calories, then you are likely not in very good shape, especially if you aren't physically active.

The sad truth in my experience is this is the way many people eat every day. Some substitute an unhealthy breakfast in place of no breakfast (adding more empty calories) but the results are still the same. So what did I do instead of my usual no breakfast and random lunch and dinner?

I started substituting 2 meals (with my meal replacement shakes), usually breakfast and lunch, but sometimes breakfast and dinner. Early in the process, it definitely took discipline for me to stick with my shakes because even though I was full in the sense that I was getting everything I was supposed to get in a full meal, I didn't have that tight stomach feeling that we associate with being full.

It took me a couple of weeks to get used to that feeling, but being able to eat the foods I wanted to eat on my 3rd meal (my non replacement meal) helped me to get used to it all very quickly. Honestly, if the plan would have required me to completely cut out all of the foods I like, then the program wouldn't have been worth it to me. I am not a body builder nor am I a fitness model. I just want to be healthy and look pretty good.

If a person really wants to change their health, physique, or both, they will have to apply discipline to some area of their lives. The question is would that person rather apply that discipline to not ever eating the foods they really like or if they prefer to apply that discipline to replacing two meals a day until it becomes a part of their lifestyle.

Which would you choose?

The End

www.ingramcontent.com/pod-product-compliance
Lightning Source LLC
Chambersburg PA
CBHW050049260726
48658CB00005B/1854